WELLNESS
journal

....

START DATE: ....

WEIGHT: ....

MEASUREMENTS:

NECK ....

SHOULDERS ....

CHEST ....

BICEP ....

WAIST ....

HIPS ....

THIGH ....

KNEE ....

CALF ....

Cover vector by Rawpixel/Freepik
Copyright © Now Paper Goods

No portion of this publication may be reproduced or transmitted in any form or by any means, electronic or mechanical, including, but not limited to, audio recordings, facsimiles, photocopying, or information storage and retrieval systems without explicit written permission from the author or publisher.

"The best project you'll ever work on is YOU."

WELLNESS goals

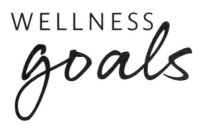

Choose goals that are realistic and achievable but require you to step out of your comfort zone.

Setting **SMART** goals will help you succeed. Consider the following SMART guidelines when choosing your wellness goals. Good luck!

S.M.A.R.T goal setting guidelines:

Be **Specific**. Describe your goal in detail.
Make it **Measurable**. How will you know when the goal is completed?
Your goal should be **Achievable**. What steps can you take?
Be **Realistic**. Do you have the right commitment and resources?
Set a **Timely** goal, with a start and finish date, to stay motivated.

GOAL ONE:
....
....

THIS GOAL IS IMPORTANT TO ME BECAUSE:
....

STEPS TO COMPLETE THIS GOAL:
....
....
....

DATE I WILL ACHIEVE THIS GOAL BY:
....

WHEN I ACHIEVE MY GOAL, MY LIFE WILL IMPROVE IN THE FOLLOWING WAYS:
....
....

IF I COMPLETE THIS GOAL BY MY TARGET DATE I WILL REWARD MYSELF WITH:
....

GOAL TWO:

THIS GOAL IS IMPORTANT TO ME BECAUSE:

STEPS TO COMPLETE THIS GOAL:

DATE I WILL ACHIEVE THIS GOAL BY:

WHEN I ACHIEVE MY GOAL, MY LIFE WILL IMPROVE IN THE FOLLOWING WAYS:

IF I COMPLETE THIS GOAL BY MY TARGET DATE I WILL REWARD MYSELF WITH:

GOAL THREE:

THIS GOAL IS IMPORTANT TO ME BECAUSE:

STEPS TO COMPLETE THIS GOAL:

DATE I WILL ACHIEVE THIS GOAL BY:

WHEN I ACHIEVE MY GOAL, MY LIFE WILL IMPROVE IN THE FOLLOWING WAYS:

IF I COMPLETE THIS GOAL BY MY TARGET DATE I WILL REWARD MYSELF WITH:

EXERCISE

WEEK 1: _____

	ACTIVITY	TIME
MONDAY		
TUESDAY		
WEDNESDAY		
THURSDAY		
FRIDAY		
SATURDAY		
SUNDAY		

This week's focus:

DISTANCE	SETS	REPS	WEIGHT

FOOD

WEEK 1: _____

	MONDAY	TUESDAY	WEDNESDAY
BREAKFAST			
LUNCH			
DINNER			
SNACKS			
WATER	○○○○ ○○○○	○○○○ ○○○○	○○○○ ○○○○
OTHER BEVERAGES			
NOTES			

This week's focus:

THURSDAY	FRIDAY	SATURDAY	SUNDAY
٥٥٥٥ ٥٥٥٥	٥٥٥٥ ٥٥٥٥	٥٥٥٥ ٥٥٥٥	٥٥٥٥ ٥٥٥٥

WELLNESS

WEEK 1: _____

	MONDAY	TUESDAY	WEDNESDAY
HOURS SLEPT/TIME			
WOKE UP FEELING...			
MOOD			
ENERGY			
PAIN			
STRESS/ ANXIETY			
TODAY'S ACTIVITIES			

This week's focus:

THURSDAY	FRIDAY	SATURDAY	SUNDAY

NOTES

WEEK 1

EXERCISE

WEEK 2:

	ACTIVITY	TIME
MONDAY		
TUESDAY		
WEDNESDAY		
THURSDAY		
FRIDAY		
SATURDAY		
SUNDAY		

This week's focus:

DISTANCE	SETS	REPS	WEIGHT

FOOD

WEEK 2: _____

	MONDAY	TUESDAY	WEDNESDAY
BREAKFAST			
LUNCH			
DINNER			
SNACKS			
WATER	○○○○ ○○○○	○○○○ ○○○○	○○○○ ○○○○
OTHER BEVERAGES			
NOTES			

This week's focus:

THURSDAY	FRIDAY	SATURDAY	SUNDAY
○○○○ ○○○○	○○○○ ○○○○	○○○○ ○○○○	○○○○ ○○○○

WELLNESS

WEEK 2: _____

	MONDAY	TUESDAY	WEDNESDAY
HOURS SLEPT/TIME			
WOKE UP FEELING…			
MOOD			
ENERGY			
PAIN			
STRESS/ ANXIETY			
TODAY'S ACTIVITIES			

This week's focus:

THURSDAY	FRIDAY	SATURDAY	SUNDAY

NOTES

WEEK 2

EXERCISE

WEEK 3: _____

	ACTIVITY	TIME
MONDAY		
TUESDAY		
WEDNESDAY		
THURSDAY		
FRIDAY		
SATURDAY		
SUNDAY		

This week's focus:

DISTANCE	SETS	REPS	WEIGHT

FOOD

WEEK 3: _____

	MONDAY	TUESDAY	WEDNESDAY
BREAKFAST			
LUNCH			
DINNER			
SNACKS			
WATER	○○○○ ○○○○	○○○○ ○○○○	○○○○ ○○○○
OTHER BEVERAGES			
NOTES			

This week's focus:

THURSDAY	FRIDAY	SATURDAY	SUNDAY
○○○○ ○○○○	○○○○ ○○○○	○○○○ ○○○○	○○○○ ○○○○

WELLNESS

WEEK 3: _____

	MONDAY	TUESDAY	WEDNESDAY
HOURS SLEPT/TIME			
WOKE UP FEELING...			
MOOD			
ENERGY			
PAIN			
STRESS/ANXIETY			
TODAY'S ACTIVITIES			

This week's focus:

THURSDAY	FRIDAY	SATURDAY	SUNDAY

NOTES

WEEK 3

EXERCISE

WEEK 4: _____

	ACTIVITY	TIME
MONDAY		
TUESDAY		
WEDNESDAY		
THURSDAY		
FRIDAY		
SATURDAY		
SUNDAY		

This week's focus:

DISTANCE	SETS	REPS	WEIGHT

FOOD

WEEK 4: _____

	MONDAY	TUESDAY	WEDNESDAY
BREAKFAST			
LUNCH			
DINNER			
SNACKS			
WATER	○○○○ ○○○○	○○○○ ○○○○	○○○○ ○○○○
OTHER BEVERAGES			
NOTES			

This week's focus:

THURSDAY	FRIDAY	SATURDAY	SUNDAY
○○○○ ○○○○	○○○○ ○○○○	○○○○ ○○○○	○○○○ ○○○○

WELLNESS

WEEK 4: ─────────

	MONDAY	TUESDAY	WEDNESDAY
HOURS SLEPT/TIME			
WOKE UP FEELING...			
MOOD			
ENERGY			
PAIN			
STRESS/ ANXIETY			
TODAY'S ACTIVITIES			

This week's focus:

THURSDAY	FRIDAY	SATURDAY	SUNDAY

NOTES

WEEK 4

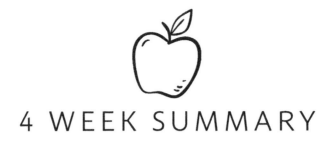

4 WEEK SUMMARY

DATE: ....

WEIGHT: ....

MEASUREMENTS:

NECK ....

SHOULDERS ....

CHEST ....

BICEP ....

WAIST ....

HIPS ....

THIGH ....

KNEE ....

CALF ....

NOTES:
....
....
....
....
....
....
....
....
....

"When you feel like giving up, remember why you started."

EXERCISE

WEEK 5: _____

	ACTIVITY	TIME
MONDAY		
TUESDAY		
WEDNESDAY		
THURSDAY		
FRIDAY		
SATURDAY		
SUNDAY		

This week's focus:

DISTANCE	SETS	REPS	WEIGHT

FOOD

WEEK 5: _____

	MONDAY	TUESDAY	WEDNESDAY
BREAKFAST			
LUNCH			
DINNER			
SNACKS			
WATER			
OTHER BEVERAGES			
NOTES			

This week's focus:

THURSDAY	FRIDAY	SATURDAY	SUNDAY
○○○○ ○○○○	○○○○ ○○○○	○○○○ ○○○○	○○○○ ○○○○

WELLNESS

WEEK 5: _____

	MONDAY	TUESDAY	WEDNESDAY
HOURS SLEPT/TIME			
WOKE UP FEELING...			
MOOD			
ENERGY			
PAIN			
STRESS/ ANXIETY			
TODAY'S ACTIVITIES			

This week's focus:

THURSDAY	FRIDAY	SATURDAY	SUNDAY

NOTES

WEEK 5

EXERCISE

WEEK 6: _____

	ACTIVITY	TIME
MONDAY		
TUESDAY		
WEDNESDAY		
THURSDAY		
FRIDAY		
SATURDAY		
SUNDAY		

This week's focus:

DISTANCE	SETS	REPS	WEIGHT

FOOD

WEEK 6: _____

	MONDAY	TUESDAY	WEDNESDAY
BREAKFAST			
LUNCH			
DINNER			
SNACKS			
WATER	○○○○ ○○○○	○○○○ ○○○○	○○○○ ○○○○
OTHER BEVERAGES			
NOTES			

This week's focus:

THURSDAY	FRIDAY	SATURDAY	SUNDAY
○○○○ ○○○○	○○○○ ○○○○	○○○○ ○○○○	○○○○ ○○○○

WELLNESS

WEEK 6: _____

	MONDAY	TUESDAY	WEDNESDAY
HOURS SLEPT/TIME			
WOKE UP FEELING…			
MOOD			
ENERGY			
PAIN			
STRESS/ ANXIETY			
TODAY'S ACTIVITIES			

This week's focus:

THURSDAY	FRIDAY	SATURDAY	SUNDAY

NOTES

WEEK 6

EXERCISE

WEEK 7:

	ACTIVITY	TIME
MONDAY		
TUESDAY		
WEDNESDAY		
THURSDAY		
FRIDAY		
SATURDAY		
SUNDAY		

This week's focus:

DISTANCE	SETS	REPS	WEIGHT

FOOD

WEEK 7: _____

	MONDAY	TUESDAY	WEDNESDAY
BREAKFAST			
LUNCH			
DINNER			
SNACKS			
WATER	○○○○ ○○○○	○○○○ ○○○○	○○○○ ○○○○
OTHER BEVERAGES			
NOTES			

This week's focus:

THURSDAY	FRIDAY	SATURDAY	SUNDAY
◌◌◌◌ ◌◌◌◌	◌◌◌◌ ◌◌◌◌	◌◌◌◌ ◌◌◌◌	◌◌◌◌ ◌◌◌◌

WELLNESS

WEEK 7: _____

	MONDAY	TUESDAY	WEDNESDAY
HOURS SLEPT/TIME			
WOKE UP FEELING...			
MOOD			
ENERGY			
PAIN			
STRESS/ ANXIETY			
TODAY'S ACTIVITIES			

This week's focus:

THURSDAY	FRIDAY	SATURDAY	SUNDAY

NOTES

WEEK 7

EXERCISE

WEEK 8: _____

	ACTIVITY	TIME
MONDAY		
TUESDAY		
WEDNESDAY		
THURSDAY		
FRIDAY		
SATURDAY		
SUNDAY		

This week's focus:

DISTANCE	SETS	REPS	WEIGHT

FOOD

WEEK 8: _____

	MONDAY	TUESDAY	WEDNESDAY
BREAKFAST			
LUNCH			
DINNER			
SNACKS			
WATER	○○○○ ○○○○	○○○○ ○○○○	○○○○ ○○○○
OTHER BEVERAGES			
NOTES			

This week's focus:

THURSDAY	FRIDAY	SATURDAY	SUNDAY
○○○○ ○○○○	○○○○ ○○○○	○○○○ ○○○○	○○○○ ○○○○

WELLNESS

WEEK 8: _____

	MONDAY	TUESDAY	WEDNESDAY
HOURS SLEPT/TIME			
WOKE UP FEELING...			
MOOD			
ENERGY			
PAIN			
STRESS/ ANXIETY			
TODAY'S ACTIVITIES			

This week's focus:

THURSDAY	FRIDAY	SATURDAY	SUNDAY

NOTES

WEEK 8

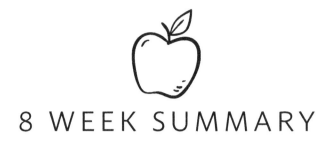

8 WEEK SUMMARY

DATE: ....

WEIGHT: ....

MEASUREMENTS:

NECK ....

SHOULDERS ....

CHEST ....

BICEP ....

WAIST ....

HIPS ....

THIGH ....

KNEE ....

CALF ....

NOTES:
....
....
....
....
....
....
....
....

> "If it doesn't challenge you it won't change you."

EXERCISE

WEEK 9:

	ACTIVITY	TIME
MONDAY		
TUESDAY		
WEDNESDAY		
THURSDAY		
FRIDAY		
SATURDAY		
SUNDAY		

This week's focus:

DISTANCE	SETS	REPS	WEIGHT

FOOD

WEEK 9: _____

	MONDAY	TUESDAY	WEDNESDAY
BREAKFAST			
LUNCH			
DINNER			
SNACKS			
WATER	○○○○ ○○○○	○○○○ ○○○○	○○○○ ○○○○
OTHER BEVERAGES			
NOTES			

This week's focus:

THURSDAY	FRIDAY	SATURDAY	SUNDAY
○○○○ ○○○○	○○○○ ○○○○	○○○○ ○○○○	○○○○ ○○○○

WELLNESS

WEEK 9: _____

	MONDAY	TUESDAY	WEDNESDAY
HOURS SLEPT/TIME			
WOKE UP FEELING...			
MOOD			
ENERGY			
PAIN			
STRESS/ ANXIETY			
TODAY'S ACTIVITIES			

This week's focus:

THURSDAY	FRIDAY	SATURDAY	SUNDAY

NOTES

WEEK 9

EXERCISE

WEEK 10: _____

	ACTIVITY	TIME
MONDAY		
TUESDAY		
WEDNESDAY		
THURSDAY		
FRIDAY		
SATURDAY		
SUNDAY		

This week's focus:

DISTANCE	SETS	REPS	WEIGHT

FOOD

WEEK 10: _____

	MONDAY	TUESDAY	WEDNESDAY
BREAKFAST			
LUNCH			
DINNER			
SNACKS			
WATER	○○○○ ○○○○	○○○○ ○○○○	○○○○ ○○○○
OTHER BEVERAGES			
NOTES			

This week's focus:

THURSDAY	FRIDAY	SATURDAY	SUNDAY
◊◊◊◊ ◊◊◊◊	◊◊◊◊ ◊◊◊◊	◊◊◊◊ ◊◊◊◊	◊◊◊◊ ◊◊◊◊

WELLNESS

WEEK 10: _____

	MONDAY	TUESDAY	WEDNESDAY
HOURS SLEPT/TIME			
WOKE UP FEELING...			
MOOD			
ENERGY			
PAIN			
STRESS/ ANXIETY			
TODAY'S ACTIVITIES			

This week's focus:

THURSDAY	FRIDAY	SATURDAY	SUNDAY

NOTES

WEEK 10

EXERCISE

WEEK 11: _____

	ACTIVITY	TIME
MONDAY		
TUESDAY		
WEDNESDAY		
THURSDAY		
FRIDAY		
SATURDAY		
SUNDAY		

This week's focus:

DISTANCE	SETS	REPS	WEIGHT

FOOD

WEEK 11: _____

	MONDAY	TUESDAY	WEDNESDAY
BREAKFAST			
LUNCH			
DINNER			
SNACKS			
WATER			
OTHER BEVERAGES			
NOTES			

This week's focus:

THURSDAY	FRIDAY	SATURDAY	SUNDAY
◊◊◊◊ ◊◊◊◊	◊◊◊◊ ◊◊◊◊	◊◊◊◊ ◊◊◊◊	◊◊◊◊ ◊◊◊◊

WELLNESS

WEEK 11: _____

	MONDAY	TUESDAY	WEDNESDAY
HOURS SLEPT/TIME			
WOKE UP FEELING…			
MOOD			
ENERGY			
PAIN			
STRESS/ANXIETY			
TODAY'S ACTIVITIES			

This week's focus:

THURSDAY	FRIDAY	SATURDAY	SUNDAY

NOTES

WEEK 11

EXERCISE

WEEK 12: _____

	ACTIVITY	TIME
MONDAY		
TUESDAY		
WEDNESDAY		
THURSDAY		
FRIDAY		
SATURDAY		
SUNDAY		

This week's focus:

DISTANCE	SETS	REPS	WEIGHT

FOOD

WEEK 12: _____

	MONDAY	TUESDAY	WEDNESDAY
BREAKFAST			
LUNCH			
DINNER			
SNACKS			
WATER	○○○○ ○○○○	○○○○ ○○○○	○○○○ ○○○○
OTHER BEVERAGES			
NOTES			

This week's focus:

THURSDAY	FRIDAY	SATURDAY	SUNDAY
○○○○ ○○○○	○○○○ ○○○○	○○○○ ○○○○	○○○○ ○○○○

WELLNESS

WEEK 12: _____

	MONDAY	TUESDAY	WEDNESDAY
HOURS SLEPT/TIME			
WOKE UP FEELING…			
MOOD			
ENERGY			
PAIN			
STRESS/ANXIETY			
TODAY'S ACTIVITIES			

This week's focus:

THURSDAY	FRIDAY	SATURDAY	SUNDAY

NOTES

WEEK 12

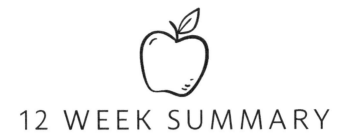

12 WEEK SUMMARY

DATE: ....

WEIGHT: ....

MEASUREMENTS:

NECK ....

SHOULDERS ....

CHEST ....

BICEP ....

WAIST ....

HIPS ....

THIGH ....

KNEE ....

CALF ....

NOTES:

....
....
....
....
....
....
....
....
....

"Keep going,
keep growing."

Made in the USA
Coppell, TX
11 March 2020